THE
HOSPICE
DECISION

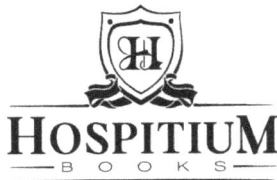

HOSPITIUM
B O O K S

Published by
HospitiuM Books
An Imprint of HospitiuM Media
HospitiumUSA.org

Houston

THE
HOSPICE
DECISION

GET PROACTIVE, FIND PERSPECTIVE, AND LIVE YOUR FULLEST LIFE

RANDAL J. SALYER, RN

for Seth and Samantha

Disclaimer

This book does not offer any medical advice. People are vastly different and medical situations have more variables than could ever be enumerated. There is no substitute for real time analysis of your current situation by the professionals involved in your unique case. The Hospice Decision must only be made by patients and families after considering medical advice and prognoses from their individual providers, against the backdrop of their own beliefs and cultural and social mores, tempered by their personal preferences and goals.

This book is an offering of my neighborly but experienced opinion. The information herein is, in my opinion, well-reasoned and formulated by keen observation at the bedsides of hundreds of patients. This is what I would, and do teach my family and friends.

The statements in this book are true to the best of my knowledge at the time of this writing but an endeavor like this is daunting, as it's impossible to account for every scenario, and things change. Things at the crossroads of government and healthcare are especially subject to change. Any mention of government or other regulation, public policy, or private agency policy, is intended to be a broad, overly simplified statement to illustrate a larger point about how or why something might or might not be done by your hospice agency. This brings us full circle to the basic point of this disclaimer, which is to say, this book is my opinion.

The point of this work is to help you develop the right mindset, gain the right perspective, and to be able to confidently use the resources that are available to you for the best possible end of life experience.

Contents

Acknowledgements

Mom and Dad, I could never have synthesized this or any other information without the foundation you provided through your wisdom, example, and teaching.

Lisa, Andy, Jeff, Julie and Royden, Each of you has impacted my life in so many positive ways I can neither recount nor repay them.

Stephanie, Every day I marvel at what you contribute to my life and to our family.

Special Thanks to:
Mr. Brian Hegvold for rescuing my graphics.
Mrs. Judy Servidio for your insight which led to a significant addition.
David Braidic for your support of this project and your friendship.
Dad, for your tireless editing despite your own exhausting list.
Seth Salyer, for your supportive interest, and for being an indispensable utility player on this project.

I would also like to acknowledge the numerous families I have been privileged to serve which knew, either intuitively or through deliberate study of life and mortality, how to have a warm and enriching end of life experience. This work was inspired by you.

Foreword

One of the most difficult situations in the ER is the terminally ill patient that is near death, brought in by distraught and anxious family members. The family hasn't been mentally or emotionally prepared and often just wants "everything done" for their loved one but the patient really shouldn't be further traumatized by futile treatments in a stressful and cold ER. There is a better way. Many think of the Hospice Decision as "giving up" so it's often not discussed when it should be. However, hospice care is not as much about dying as it is about peaceful living to the end.

Julie Morgan M.D.
Emergency Physician

So teach us to number our days, that we may apply our hearts unto wisdom.—Psalm 90:12

Introduction

I love that moment. There's a recurring moment in dealing with hospice families that keeps me doing what I do. There's almost always a moment when a family caregiver's shoulders drop…

I can't tell you how often I've walked into a home where a hospice diagnosis was still fresh. The anxiety is so intense as patients and families minds are reeling, trying desperately to come to terms with what they've just been told. "What does it all mean?" "How will we proceed?" "How will this affect our resources?" "How will I deal with my feelings?" "How will we tell the family?" "I can't believe I'm hearing the word hospice." "What does that really mean?" "What will hospice do for us?"

Usually, people are so tense that they don't realize that they have stopped breathing deeply. Their shoulders are up around their ears. I remember well, dealing with a lady of retirement age who was the primary caregiver for her mom. This lady was very stressed out about caring for her mother. Not knowing what to expect, she was so on edge that every time my necessary but subtle, and very quiet email chimed from my cell phone in my shirt pocket, she nearly jumped out of her chair. It happened more than once. Her hands would come up to shoulder level, palms down, fingers out. Her knees drove her ankles backward so that her legs rested on the balls of her feet as if she were poised to spring into action. Despite still sitting at the kitchen table, her body had morphed into what looked like a basketball player's defensive position.

All this anxiety came from uncertainty. It came from a lack of understanding of what to expect and how to proceed.

So many times I've walked into houses with similar scenarios. But this is the whole reason I work in hospice. Sometimes people hear what I do and say "Oh, that must be terribly depressing." But they don't know what I know-- that so often I've been able to go into a home that is under a pall of anxiety and helplessness and fear, and change that environment. Where families and patients are accepting of help, I have been able to speak honestly with them and to give them truth openly. I've been able to answer their questions and help them understand what's happening and what to expect. I've been able to help them understand the process of their particular disease and the process of death and dying. And maybe most important, I have been able to dissuade that feeling of helplessness by giving them a plan. This includes teaching them how to intervene when symptoms arise or how and when to call for help. And then there's the crux of why I do this work. It's the moment in hospice that I live for. I love that moment when the anxiety starts to evaporate, and the fear begins to fade into the past. It's that moment when the teaching, and the confidence in my voice, and the reassurance of having a plan, and knowing they are not alone begins to unravel that tension. Then, there it is. The first, big, deep cleansing breath they've breathed in a long time. At that moment there is new resolve. They begin to relax. I live for that moment when their shoulders drop.

I share this moment with people almost on a daily basis. And while outsiders think it must be terribly depressing, I find it to be profoundly positive and uplifting.

Traditionally, our healthcare system is very much focused on fixing problems. And our ever increasingly urban society has become disturbingly insulated from death. We want to ignore it, pretend it doesn't exist. We want to bury our heads in the sand until we're absolutely forced to face it. But the reality is that medical science, for all of its advancements, cannot fix everything. Certainly, the cycle of life does not need to be fixed. The mortality rate for human beings has always been and will always be 100%. Death is as much a part of life as birth is a part of life. They are two ends of the same spectrum. But human beings have the capacity to die well with grace and dignity.

I wrote this book in high hopes that people everywhere, facing the end of life, both patients, and caregivers, would be able to embrace that capacity of humans to die well. I hope that in these pages you will find within yourself, the ability to gain the perspective that you need to move forward with a profound peace. It's also my sincere desire that after reading this book, you will understand what hospice is and what it can do for you. So take a deep cleansing breath. Accept a new resolve, and proceed with confidence.

SECTION I

TWO JOURNEYS

A Fable

The 1987 Cutlass Supreme turned down Seventh Avenue as it had done so many times before. But today there was a melancholy shadow looming over the car. The passenger seat in the old Cutlass was comfortable. Hank had reclined slightly and positioned himself so that his weight was mostly resting on his right hip. His right hand pulled down slightly on the upper part of the seat belt to keep it from digging into his neck. Throughout the entire trip home from the hospital, Hank never broke his gaze. He peered past the vibrating raindrops on his side window. The sites were familiar now; they were almost home. As they passed Jim's house, Hank didn't know exactly what he was feeling, but he knew that he was affected in some way by the scene in Jim's front yard. Jim's grandkids were playing on the swing that Jim had hung from the massive oak tree that shaded his house. "Jim's life always seems so perfect," Hank thought to himself.

Hank was angry. His doctor hadn't been very empathetic when he delivered the news of Hank's poor prognosis and short life expectancy. To make matters worse, the hospital had bungled his discharge, leaving him waiting in a cold hallway for 2 hours. Hank's sister Liz, who was driving the car had been going on and on, about the debacle with the delivery of the medical equipment to their house, not seeming to notice Hank's lack of response.

Intellectually, Liz understood what was happening to Hank, but emotionally she never accepted his poor prognosis. She certainly did not buy into the concept of end-of-life care. Hank and Liz had been through a lot together. They'd had each other's backs through the many misfortunes that life had dealt them. When they were kids, they called themselves the "dynamic duo." The adults in the neighborhood just called them "partners in crime." After all they had been through together, Liz felt that participating in end-of-life care was like giving up on Hank.

Liz's perspective was not a good combination with Hank's anger. Without ever consciously intending it, their respective outlooks worked in concert to revive the old dynamic duo, but now under the fog of Hank's disease, their partnership had a new element of bitterness. This time they were united against the world.

Hank and Liz had both listened quietly when the hospice people came to talk to them at the hospital. The idea of having some help with Hank's care was attractive to them. They were especially happy to hear that someone would be coming to help Hank with his bathing since he was having more difficulty with that lately, and Liz was worried about his safety. It also sounded like the hospice agency was going to provide a lot of equipment, things they knew they needed but didn't know how they were going to pay for. So they signed the papers giving their consent to be treated by hospice.

But while they allowed the hospice agency to provide some services, they never actually faced the truth of Hank's illness--that he was dying. They weren't open to the truth. And because of that, they never processed what was happening. They never stepped back to clarify their goals. Instead, they built a wall of illusion around themselves. Or, perhaps it was delusion. The delusion was the idea that by controlling the things and people around them, somehow they could control the outcome of Hank's disease.

Instead of allowing hospice to really help them, they reinforced their delusion. They clung to anything that gave them the sense that they were in control. They made demands and created impossible standards. When their demands couldn't be fulfilled, or their standards met, they became frustrated and angry. Feeling angry or frustrated actually gave them a short term satisfaction. It made them feel justified. It validated in their own minds that they had been right all along.

They regularly disregarded instructions from the hospice care providers and took the management of Hank's care into their own hands. They used the medications that hospice provided, but they tinkered with the doses. They supplemented their medication regimen with a lot of over the counter medications without ever mentioning the additions to the hospice nurse.

Hank's unsatisfactory demise came as a result of a crucial miscalculation on his part. Over a period of several days, Hank's condition had deteriorated significantly. The hospice nurse had tried on more than one occasion to explain to Liz and Hank that Hank was in a new phase of decline. She carefully and patiently outlined the process of Hank's disease. She talked about the symptoms that they might expect.

The nurse sat at the bedside and opened the little cardboard box that had been provided by the hospice. They called it the comfort kit. It was a collection of 6 or 7 different types of medications. These medications weren't intended to be taken regularly, but the hospice kept them in the home to manage symptoms that are common at the end of life. The nurse felt that Hank was beginning to enter the final phase of his disease and she wanted to make sure that they, Liz in particular, understood how and when to use the medications. She pulled them out of the box, one at a time, and explained what each one was called and what it was used for. She explained how to spot the symptoms and how each medication should be administered. Hank and Liz were only half listening. Why should they listen? After all, they had convinced themselves that the hospice had failed them at every step. The nurse asked Liz to repeat the instructions, just to be sure that she understood, but Liz declined to do so. She said, "No that's okay, I got it." Before the nurse left, she asked Hank and Liz if they had any questions, but neither did. The nurse said, "Okay, well you can call us anytime if you have questions, or if something changes."

About two hours had passed since the nurse left the home. Hank's symptoms were getting worse. Because Hank had taken his medications inconsistently at best, and not at all according to directions, none of the medications that the hospice gave them seemed to him to be working. Later that evening, Hank's symptoms became so bad that he made the decision to have

Liz drive him to the hospital, once again ignoring the nurse's instructions.

Hank and Liz sat in the waiting room of the emergency room for almost two hours. When they finally called Hank back to a room, a nurse came in immediately to ask what was going on, but it was quite sometime after that when they finally saw the doctor. Hank's pain was really starting to get out of control now. Liz tried to explain the situation to the doctor and nurses at the emergency room. "I don't understand it", she said. "He has taken everything the hospice has given him."

"Oh, I see," said the doctor. "How long has he been a hospice patient?" The doctor pulled the stethoscope from around his neck and stepped toward Hank.

"It's been about three months, I guess," Liz said. The doctor continued his examination without responding.

"So, tell me what medications has Hank taken today?" The doctor was trying to figure out how he could help. He had directed the question to Liz, but his body language made it clear that he was looking for either one of them to answer.

By now, Hank was in too much pain, and too frustrated to answer. Liz tried, but she honestly didn't know for sure. There hadn't been much rhyme or reason to how Hank had taken his medicine. He had pretty much taken whatever he thought he needed, whenever he thought he needed it.

"Well, I know he's been taking morphine."

"Okay", said the doctor, sensing Liz's hesitation, "how much and how often?"

"I guess I don't really know", she stammered. "He kind of just…takes it."

The doctor realized that he wasn't going to get much

information directly from Hank and Liz, and he excused himself. "Alright, you two don't go anywhere. We're going to start an I.V. and get him something for that pain. I'm going to check into his medical records, and then we'll talk."

The doctor caught one of the nurses in the hallway and had him start an I.V. and then he wrote an order for a cautious dose of morphine.

About twenty-five minutes had gone by when the doctor slid open the sliding glass door and stepped back into Hank's room. The morphine had begun to take the edge off of the pain. The doctor rolled the little exam stool out from under the sink and sat down. He took his glasses off and folded them and tucked them into the pocket protector in his lab coat. "Hank," he said, "I've read your medical history thoroughly. And you know it's quite extensive." Hank and Liz were silent. "I'm sure it's not news to you that—medically speaking—you have an awful lot of things going on." He went on. "I see where Dr. Morgan had a pretty lengthy discussion with you regarding hospice care. And Liz tells me you have been receiving hospice care for about 3 months. But I can also tell from what Liz says that you haven't been exactly cooperative with them." Liz had been standing throughout the entire visit. Now, leaning against the wall, she looked at the ground while Hank, lying in bed, stared at the ceiling. Both were avoiding eye contact with the doctor, but there was a change. They had both begun to listen. They had begun to realize that they had made a mistake in their approach. Without ever exchanging a word, they each sensed that the doctor was about to make all of this very clear to them.

"Hank, you've been dealt a lousy hand, and I'm so sorry." The doctor's tone carried an odd combination of resolve and compassion. He felt strongly that the siblings needed a firm dose of reality. This wasn't the first time he had ever had this type of discussion, not by a long shot, but it was always difficult. And while he was somewhat frustrated with Hank, that wasn't his motivation for this discussion. His motivation now was as pure as his reason for becoming a doctor in the first place—to help people. He continued, "I think you know that I'm going to tell you the same thing that Dr. Morgan did. We are not going to be able to fix the root cause of your disease. There's nothing we can do here that can't be done in your home by hospice". "The hospice can manage your symptoms and control your pain, but that will depend on you following instructions. You're going to have to start keeping records of when you take your medications and how much you're taking. That's the only way the hospice will be able to evaluate what's working and what's not." The doctor sounded strangely paternal to Hank. Strange, partly because Hank had never known his father, but also strange because the doctor, though he was no spring chicken, was clearly younger than Hank. "If you'll do that," he continued, "they'll be able to make adjustments to keep you comfortable. But I think that's where your focus should be—on staying comfortable. That way you can have the best quality of life, for whatever time you have left." Hank and Liz were still silent. The doctor added, "I'll get your discharge paperwork going so you can get home."

Hank and Liz knew that everything the doctor said was true. And for the first time, they were starting to accept the reality of Hank's condition. The doctor had even inspired them a little with his lecture. But tragically, it was too late.

When the nurse came into the room to give Hank his

discharge paperwork, Hank was starting to feel his pain increasing again. But he silently reassured himself; "I'll be home in a few minutes." He thought, "I'll get another dose of pain medicine when I get home."

As the E.R. Tech wheeled Hank out of the lobby and down the ramp toward the car, his pain intensified. With each seam in the sidewalk, Hank felt a wave of pain radiate through his body.

The ride home had been excruciating with the pain escalating moment by moment. Now, with Hank writhing in his bed, Liz decided unilaterally to call the hospice. It took the nurse about an hour to get to them. As soon as she saw Hank, she said, "Oh, Honey. What happened?" She immediately reached for the box of Morphine on Hank's bedside table and asked Liz when his last dose was.

"About an hour ago" Liz responded. "I wasn't sure what to do so we called you."

"Well, you did the right thing". The nurse said as she began to draw up another dose in the oral syringe. But as she moved the tiny syringe toward Hank, she heard Liz gasp. Only a fraction of a second later, the nurse made the same realization that Liz had. Hank had died in a crisis.

What Hank never knew was that around the corner and just three doors down, Jim, whose life Hank admired that day on the way home from the hospital, had received a similar diagnosis and life expectancy just sixteen days before Hank had received his.

Hank had met Jim on a number of occasions. The first time

they met was during their neighborhood's annual block party. The police actually came into the subdivision for that event to block off the streets to all but pedestrian traffic. Hank and Jim discovered that they shared a passion for motorcycles. They talked for a long time that night and ever since then they had always made an effort to speak to one another at the neighborhood watch meetings which they both attended religiously.

Hank was careful to project an air of equality with Jim in their interactions, but he was quite aware of his own feeling of inferiority. Secretly, Hank had always admired Jim's life. Jim was one of those guys who just always seemed to have it all together. And, while Hank had always felt a little lonely, it didn't escape him that Jim always seemed to have visitors' cars in the driveway. He certainly noticed the grandkids playing in the yard every weekend.

Like Hank, Jim had encountered numerous frustrations surrounding his care and treatments. There was a period of time at the hospital when it seemed that nothing went according to plan. And Jim too had experiences with doctors and nurses that had left a sour taste in his mouth. But despite the uncanny similarities in the two men's situations, there was a stark difference in their approach. Jim's outlook and demeanor embodied what Robert Frost was writing about in "The Road Not Taken"; Jim took the less traveled road and indeed, it made all the difference.

When Jim received the news of his diagnosis and short life expectancy he embarked on a profound personal journey. It was not a journey of a geographical nature. It was a journey of discovery. Jim traveled the oft-neglected neuropathways of higher thought. He wrestled with God, and he wrestled with the great issues of life.

Immediately after Jim had gotten his diagnosis of the terminal disease, he still had quite a lot of functional ability. He wasn't having symptoms, and he really didn't feel all that bad, but his mind was reeling. Throughout his life though, Jim had developed the ability to get inside his own head whenever he needed to gain perspective or make a major decision. This time was no exception. He knew exactly what he needed to do.

The drive to Crystal Lake was not easy with its winding roads and steep elevation gain. But that leg of the trip seemed almost ceremonial to Jim. It was like the preamble to the poetry of his escape. Of course, he wasn't fleeing responsibility, on the contrary, he was escaping the noise and bustle of the city, and the routines of his life precisely so that he could mentally process the realities he faced. The payoff of the challenging drive was the solitude he found among the tall pines. The heavy silence of the woods was interrupted only by the breeze rustling the leaves or the chatter of a chipmunk. This place had become the primary destination of what had been a semi-regular pilgrimage for Jim in his life's decisions and struggles.

Over the years, Jim had cultivated this practice. He learned to ask himself specific questions that helped him prioritize his thoughts and values. Jim wedged himself into a cleft in a huge fallen tree and unwrapped the laces of his leather-bound journal. He actually kept a written list of these questions and used them as a matrix to sort his thoughts and priorities any time he was facing a significant fork in his life's road.

Jim had arranged the questions in his journal in such a way as to facilitate the free flow of deep thinking. The first question was important but non-threatening. It simply said,

"What have been my life's happiest memories, and why?"

This opened the floodgates of Jim's mind. His senses erupted. He remembered a fishing trip with his dad when he was just a young boy. His heart rate picked up a little as he recalled the excitement he felt in anticipation of that trip. He didn't perceive it, but Jim had begun to smile. He thought about how carefree he had been then, and how at that time, his life was so pure and basic. He remembered another time when his family found an abandoned nest of baby rabbits. It had been a whole-family project. They nursed them along, keeping them in a shoebox. Jim's memory of the event was so powerful that it was as if he could actually smell the cedar chips they had used to line the bottom of the shoebox. Memories were still flowing. He remembered the day he met his wife. That thought was quickly followed by the memory of the moment he realized he was going to marry her. He thought about the early years of their marriage when they had nothing. He remembered one day in particular, an afternoon they spent building bookshelves with borrowed tools and scrap lumber. They had cranked up the radio and were singing along and sharing a single bottle of beer. He remembered the births of each of his children and teaching them skills like riding bikes and working with wood. He thought about the significant milestones of each of his kids. He remembered the first time he became a grandfather and how it was such a different experience than having his own children had been.

Jim settled even further into the cleft in the tree. He leaned back and closed his eyes. He felt the sun coming through the forest canopy and warming his face. He let out a big sigh and basked for a moment in the collection of those memories.

He started to feel grounded in that moment. He was already gaining a perspective of what was important to him which led seamlessly to the next question:

"What are the 3 most important things in my life?"

Jim didn't deliberate. He just embraced the first things that came to his mind. They actually entered his consciousness in order of priority. "My faith", he thought. "My marriage"…"my kids." It almost seemed too easy. It seemed like a question of this gravity should demand more time and effort. "Maybe I've got it wrong", Jim thought. "After all, I am in the middle of a health crisis. That's why I'm here in the first place. Why hadn't that entered into my head?" he asked himself. "People always say 'well, at least I've got my health' as if that's of paramount importance and it always rang true" Jim searched his answers again, but as he thought it through, he reaffirmed his initial response. He had built his whole life around his faith. It was much bigger than his own life. It was the prism through which he viewed everything, including his new diagnosis. His relationship with his wife had been established through that faith, and together they built a marriage that emanated from those shared values. They had worked so hard to pass their faith and values on to their children, and to develop a strong family identity around those concepts. Jim was starting to feel a deep sense of clarity now. He was confident in the validity of his priorities. With his core values in mind, Jim proceeded to the third question.

"What do I want to accomplish in my life?"

It was a question that Jim had asked himself so many times before, but now it had taken on a whole new meaning. Before in Jim's life, when he had asked himself this question, it served to help him stay focused on major life goals. But now, in the context of his life expectancy of less than six months, this question seemed to have an essence of long range planning that wasn't quite appropriate now. Jim wanted to reframe the question. He put his head back against the tree again and closed his eyes. He thought about just reworking the question to make the tense more fitting to his current situation by asking "What have I accomplished in my life?". But he didn't see an immediate value in recounting his past accomplishments because the purpose of this retreat was to process his current situation. He drifted for a moment. With his eyes still closed, he began to absorb the sounds of the forest; the rustling of the leaves, the chatter of the squirrels in the distance, and the songbirds overhead which seemed to be having some kind of conversation. He took it all in. He inhaled deeply and smelled the pine. He opened his eyes and marveled at the way the sun's rays were visible as they shined through the trees. While he was soaking up the beauty of his surroundings, his subconscious brain was still working to determine the most appropriate question. Jim knew he needed to capture the same essence of that question, but that in his current situation, the question needed to be more specific. And it came to him. Jim unsheathed the pen from the edge of the back cover of his journal. He drew a line through the original question and wrote:

"What is the most meaningful contribution I can make to affirm my most important values?"

This question became the driving force, a mission, in the

final chapter of Jim's life. Not only did it provide a framework and perspective for his thoughts and feelings, but it provided Jim with a plan of action. It gave him a project, an end-of-life work which occupied his mind and spirit in a healthy, productive and outgoing way.

Jim knew that to guide this work, he would need to break down this overarching question into useable parts. He kept writing.

"What is the most meaningful thing I can do to affirm my faith?"

"What is the most meaningful thing I can do to affirm my marriage?"

"What is the most meaningful thing I can do to affirm my relationships with my kids?"

Jim spent another two hours in the cleft of that tree thinking, pondering, and planning his new work. When he left the woods that day, there was a spring in his step. He had a new resolve and a sharp focus. He had business to finish. And he had peace.

Because Jim had lived most of his life in the same careful, thoughtful way that had taken him to the forest that day, he also had passed on to his kids that same ability to process life's trials. When they had heard the news of Jim's diagnosis and short prognosis and that he had entered a hospice program, they too retreated to privacy to do the hard work of finding perspective.

Each in their individual ways had wrestled with their own

thoughts and feelings. And like Jim, each had to one degree or another, wrestled with God and struggled with the ultimate questions of life. And, like Jim, each had come to peace with their new reality.

Now, Jim and his family had arrived at a place of deep peace and security that they derived from their faith and from the support that they received from each other. They understood from their soul searching that death was a significant part of life.

Jim and his family had also formed a special bond with the whole hospice team. They had listened carefully to each discipline and had asked questions to tap their expertise. They had also taken the time to get to know each team member individually. They made small talk about vacations and their families, and sometimes they had more profound conversations. Each member of the hospice team felt like they had learned as much from Jim and his family through their example, as Jim and his family had learned from them.

Jim's family and close friends all gathered in during the last days of his life. Everyone contributed, each in their own way, to make Jim comfortable. They were with him—really with him.

In the final hours, there was standing room only in Jim's room. Some were perched on the sides and foot of his bed. Others were sitting on the floor. Jim's family had not only done the mental and spiritual hard work of soul searching, but they had also participated in the more physically demanding work of making sure Jim's basic needs were met and that he was comfortable.

With that foundation laid, they felt a sense of calm, empowerment and security. Now, gathered around Jim's bed they told stories and reminisced and laughed freely. Jim's grandson played the guitar while the rest of the crowd sang his favorite old country songs.

When Jim took his final breath, there were tears, but there was peace. It was a beautiful death.

This fable is just that…a fable. A fictitious story to illustrate a lesson. Fictitious though it is, I have known and personally witnessed the extreme approaches of both Hank and Jim, respectively. There's no question that the Jims of the world have a much better end of life experience.

I've watched so many people just like Hank, drive themselves and their families and caregivers to an unsatisfactory death experience because their avoidance instinct and their need to control the outcome was so strong that it ultimately dominated their thoughts and feelings and therefore dominated their perceptions, actions, and relationships.

There is perhaps an unspoken truth in our society around these scenarios. It is, that while everyone dies at some point, the end of life experience is experienced by not only the one dying, but it is experienced by all of the stakeholders, namely family, friends, and caregivers.

What the dying individual doesn't experience is what happens after the death event to all those who remain. Many times after an unsatisfactory death event, or for those who have not done the same type of thinking or end of life work that Jim did, the friends, family, and caregivers are left reeling.

Often the scenario leaves them reliving the event over and over in their minds. They struggle with questions like "Did I do something wrong?" Or "Could I have done more?". "Could or Should I have done something differently?" "Am I to blame?"

These struggles are almost always rooted in a failure of someone to realize and face mortality. Either their own or that of their dying loved one.

The realization that the end of life is a shared experience is perhaps the biggest differentiator in having an end of life experience that looks like Jim's and one that looks like Hank's.

SECTION II

DEFINING HOSPICE

What is Hospice?

DEFINITION OF HOSPICE

The word hospice is derived from the Latin hospitium meaning a place of lodging or rest for travelers. It refers to both the guest and the host.

But even the unabridged Webster's Third New International Dictionary that lies at all times, open on my credenza does not make the jump to our modern medical notion of the word. In fact, it makes no mention of any medical application at all. Instead, it refers to the concept of lodging and compares the word to our modern word hostel. This is partly why today's hospice is widely misunderstood, and the word itself has myths and stigmas swirling around it.

Many people think of hospice as a place, but this is not totally accurate. There are free-standing hospice facilities, but in the broader scope, hospice is a concept; a philosophy even. It is a holistic, interdisciplinary approach to providing comfort and quality of life, at the end of life.

Modern hospice philosophy considers the patient, the family and even close friends of the patient. It seeks to provide physical and emotional comfort to the patient but is also concerned with the psychological health and well-being of the patient's family, loved ones, and caregivers.

Hospice signifies a turning. It signifies the recognition that the end of life is near and that either medical science and its treatments can provide no further benefit to the patient, or the patient or family decides that pursuing those treatments would not be in the best interest of the patient.

The next step when that decision is made is to move toward a palliative care model. The word palliate means to cover or mask and thus, palliative care is the practice of covering or masking symptoms without intent to cure the underlying disease. Palliative care is a broad category and may be employed in a number of ways and is not always associated with a terminal diagnosis or with the last 6 months of life. Hospice is a more specific subset of palliative care, focused on providing comfort and control of symptoms in what is presumed to be the last 6 months of life.

BENEFITS OF HOSPICE

Throughout this book, we will speak of the hospice benefit. This is a more clinical term referring to payer sources, namely the Centers for Medicare and Medicaid Services among other insurance providers. But what I'm referring to now is not the insurance benefit but rather the actual or perceived benefits for you the hospice client. For the purpose of this book, the term "hospice client" will refer to anyone who benefits from the hospice service. This would include not only the patient but caregivers, family and potentially even close friends.

As a hospice client, you will receive empathetic, compassionate care by a large team working closely together with you and your family.   Hospice team nurses, doctors, social workers, chaplains, music therapists, and volunteers work together to provide comfort not only to the patient but to the patient's support system as well.

The patient will be supported medically through clinical assessments from doctors and nurses and social workers who are able to provide interventions both pharmacological and non-pharmacological, and other solutions through education and counseling. Caregivers, loved ones and family members of the patient will also receive support in the form of education, counseling, community resources as well as grief and bereavement support.

Having hospice on board means that you will have routine visitors to your home who can instruct and guide you in caring for your loved one. You will have experts you can call 24 hours a day to answer questions or even make an impromptu visit when necessary.

Hospice done right helps melt away your fears and anxiety and gives you the confidence to move forward and the peace of knowing that you're not alone.

Myths & Stigmas

MYTH: Hospice is only for cancer patients.

FACT: Hospice is for anyone that has a life expectancy of six months or less under the normal progression of the disease, regardless of the disease.

MYTH: Hospice is for those in their final hours.

FACT: Hospice is for those who are presumed to have a 6-month or less life expectancy. Because there is no science to predict how long someone will live, some hospice patients receive the hospice benefit for much longer periods of time than six months. Actually, as a hospice nurse case manager, I have experienced a great deal of frustration when a patient is not referred to hospice until they are in their final hours. It is far more beneficial for a patient to receive an earlier hospice referral which allows the hospice team to become involved and to develop a relationship with the patient and family and to help improve the quality of life for whatever time a patient has left.

MYTH: Hospice is a place.

FACT: There are dedicated inpatient hospice units, and in these cases, I suppose it could be said that the hospice is a place. Far more important to understand, is the reality that hospice is a concept and philosophy without regard to place. In fact, hospice provides care to a patient wherever the patient lives.

MYTH: Hospice facilitates death.

FACT: Hospice neither prolongs life nor hastens death. Instead, hospice works to provide comfort at the end of life.

MYTH: When the morphine is administered, death is imminent.

FACT: While it is true that morphine is often used when death is imminent, it is also used far more frequently than you might think. Morphine is an old, tried-and-true medication that is extremely useful for the reduction of moderate to severe pain. It can also be used to decrease the sensation of breathlessness in patients who are short of breath. It has the added benefit that it comes in forms and concentrations that are readily absorbed in the mouth without posing a choking hazard for patients who have difficulty swallowing. When I was under 40 years old and otherwise healthy, my appendix ruptured. Morphine was the hospital's first line of defense against my intense pain. It was very effective and did not cause my death. The mere use of morphine does not mean that death is imminent. And the use of morphine does not cause death. It is a good medication that should not be feared by patients and families when there is no allergy or documented sensitivity.

Levels of Care

There are four levels of care which hospice patients may experience. Only one type of care is applied to a patient at one time. The four distinct levels of care are outlined in the sections that follow.

1. ROUTINE CARE

Routine care is the most common level of care for a hospice patient. Routine care is provided for patients who are in the regular process of decline, where symptoms are controlled by standard measures. As with all levels of care, counseling, education, and support by the hospice team are ongoing. Routine care may be provided to a patient who is residing at home, in a long-term care facility such as a nursing home, assisted living, or board and care facility.

2. CRISIS CARE

A patient whose symptoms are not easily or adequately controlled with standard medications and therapies, or those requiring frequent medication adjustments may require crisis care, which is sometimes called continuous care. The need for this type of care will be determined by a Registered Nurse. Once the determination is made that a patient requires crisis care, the hospice agency will provide care by a licensed nurse at the bedside, around the clock or for extended periods of time within each 24-hour increment. The determination for crisis care is made in 24-hour increments. Therefore, the patient will be reassessed daily by the Nurse Case Manager or other Registered Nurse to determine whether symptoms have been adequately controlled, or whether therapies continue to require adjustment, or when the very frequent administration of medication is required to manage symptoms. The goal of care in this situation is to have the patient return to a routine level of care as soon as possible. Because of this goal, crisis care may be discontinued by the Registered Nurse at any time within each 24 hour period. It should not be expected by the family that around-the-clock crisis care at the bedside will continue indefinitely.

3. GENERAL INPATIENT CARE

General Inpatient Care is similar to crisis care in that a patient requiring general inpatient care is in need of either skilled care provided by licensed healthcare professionals on a frequent basis, or the patient is having symptoms that are not well controlled. Crisis care occurs wherever the patient is physically located. By contrast, general inpatient care only occurs where skilled professionals are available around the clock such as skilled nursing facilities dedicated inpatient hospice units and acute care hospitals. The goal of care in general inpatient status is to return the patient to the routine level of care as soon as possible.

4. RESPITE CARE

Occasionally, caregivers experience fatigue while caring for their loved one. Often in a home care setting the patient's caregiver is the only person available, day in and day out, to care for a patient. Because hospice care is directed not only toward the patient but at the patient's loved ones, hospice agencies recognize the importance of caring for families and caregivers. For this reason, hospice provides temporary placement for the patient in a skilled nursing facility for the period of five days. This five day period provides the caregiver with the opportunity to rest. Transportation of the patient to and from the skilled nursing facility may be provided by the hospice agency if the family is unable to transport the patient, for example, in the case of a bed bound patient who requires stretcher transportation.

SECTION III

THE HOSPICE JOURNEY

A Progression

Originally, I had titled this chapter "A Timeline", because people so often ask for a time-based projection. But in reality, the term timeline would be a misnomer. People are all very different, with different diseases, different histories, and different personalities. People are complex. Their situations have many variables, and therefore their timelines will vary. What follows is much more accurately thought of in terms of a progression.

DISEASE PROCESS IDENTIFIED BY PATIENT

By the time hospice comes into the picture, or the family finds itself at the crossroads of the decision to employ hospice, usually it's because the patient, at some point, has determined that there is a problem based on symptoms that he or she is having. This may seem an obvious point, but there are exceptions to this first step. Unfortunately, some people have an unexpected event while living an otherwise normal life. In one case a 65-year-old man, considered by himself and everyone who knew him, to be in exceptional health, collapsed while mowing his lawn. He never recovered consciousness. He was discovered to have a brain tumor, and the hospice decision had to be made by his family. For the purpose of this overview of a hospice journey, we will assume a slower disease progression.

DIAGNOSIS OF POTENTIAL TERMINAL DISEASE

Concerned by symptoms, the patient then follows up with his primary care physician or the ER and is subsequently diagnosed with a terminal disease. On other occasions the patient is noted by others, usually loved ones and or family members, to have some sort of deficiency. They encourage the patient to seek medical help to determine exactly what the problem is.

In more rare cases, the patient may not be aware at all that there is an underlying medical problem and it is only discovered during routine checkups or health screenings. At this time it may be possible for the terminal disease process to be treated depending on the degree to which the disease has advanced. The timing of the discovery of a terminal disease may impact the degree to which a disease can be successfully treated.

On the other hand, the disease may be well known to the patient and family, as in the case of long term chronic problems. Sometimes patients struggle for years with a disease and simply come to the point where all the known medical treatments have ceased to be effective. In these cases, the diagnosis is no surprise, but the patient and family has to shift their paradigm where treatment is concerned, from pursuing a cure to seeking comfort and quality of life.

Another factor is the goals of care of the patient and family. A patient may have already decided that they do not wish to seek curative treatment based on any number of factors including personal history, background, deeply held opinions, and religious beliefs to name a few.

Clarifying the goals of care is a powerful step in making the hospice decision. For more on this, see the chapter entitled Clarifying Goals of Care on page 95.

TREATMENT

At the time of diagnosis or immediately thereafter, a patient may elect to treat the underlying disease.

In the case of chronic diseases such as heart failure, patients may be able to sustain a relatively normal life and schedule of activities. With some chronic diseases, there is a progression of treatment in the form of medications and other interventions that the patient can go through until it is determined either by the patient or the physician that medical therapies have stopped working and can no longer be adjusted effectively.

In the case of diseases like cancer, it may be determined that a patient should go through certain treatments like chemotherapy or radiation. Sometimes even when a physician knows that these therapies will not send cancer into full remission, he might still recommend them in an effort to maximize the quality of life. This is frequently done for the relief of pain that may be caused by a tumor.

THE PHYSICIAN ENDS TREATMENT

Palliative treatments that are directed at relief of symptoms rather than directly addressing the underlying disease may continue until those treatments become ineffective (i.e., palliative chemotherapy) or when it is determined that regardless of medical treatments, a patient is nearing the end of life. At this time, a patient may be referred to hospice.

THE PATIENT OPTS OUT

Patients may also elect on their own to opt out of treatment. Sometimes this happens in the case of cancer, for instance. When a patient decides that chemotherapy or radiation or other treatment is not sufficiently adding to the quality of life and possibly is even detracting from the quality of life in such a way as to make clear the decision to cease treatments, they may decide on their own to opt out of disease-directed treatment. Often patients at this point have accepted that they are at the end of life. Hospice at this time may be a comforting option. It allows the patient or family to change gears and focus on the quality of life and care directed to comfort rather than cure.

HOSPICE REFERRAL AND SIX-MONTH PROGNOSIS

Hospice referrals are generally made by physicians when they suspect that under the normal progression of the disease, the patient's life expectancy is six months or less. I should repeat for emphasis that this is what is reasonably expected under the normal progression of the disease. This begs the question, what's normal? As with most things in life, there are too many variables to make this prediction with a great deal of accuracy. Just because it is expected to be six months or less, does not mean that it will be six months or less. Sometimes diseases are detected very late in the disease process, and therefore some patients receive the hospice benefit for a much shorter period of time.

On the other hand, because there is no science to accurately predict the moment of death, some patients will live a great deal longer than the expected six months. This can have much to do with a patient's personality. Some disease processes are known to have plateaus as in the case of congestive heart failure. Patients sometimes have a rapid decline followed by a long plateau in their condition and functional ability, followed by another decline, followed by another plateau. This cycle may continue until the patient is no longer able to sustain life.

In order for a patient to receive the hospice benefit under the Medicare Guidelines and Conditions of Participation, a physician must certify that he expects the patient to die within six months. However, Medicare recognizes that this is not a perfect science and that each individual's disease process will differ due to myriad variables, including the disease process itself, quality of care, and even the patient's personality. Therefore the initial hospice benefit period is a 90-day term. The patient can then be recertified, provided they continue to decline physically, for a second 90-day certification. After the second 90 day benefit period patients must be recertified on a 60-day basis indefinitely until the time of death. At the time of this writing, patients may receive unlimited 60-day benefits as long as a decline or progression of the disease can be demonstrated. This happens through physical exams by the RN and physician, and their subsequent documentation.

Occasionally patients will experience an upturn in their

condition whereby it is no longer presumed that they would die within a six-month period. In these cases, patients are discharged from hospice. Hospices should make every effort to connect patients with appropriate resources for ongoing healthcare. This includes the primary care provider and suppliers of durable medical equipment such as oxygen concentrators, etc., where necessary.

EXPLANATION OF BENEFITS AND BASELINE EVALUATION; DETERMINATION OF ELIGIBILITY BY NURSE

After a patient has been referred to hospice by the physician, the hospice agency makes contact with the family to set-up a meeting in which there will be an explanation of benefits. This is a sales meeting. But that's okay. It is valuable and helpful in providing the family with information regarding the services that will be provided by that particular hospice agency. You have the right to choose your hospice provider, so this is your opportunity to interview agencies. Just remember that some of these services are required by Medicare, and so all hospice agencies who accept Medicare funds will provide the same core services.

There still are, however, distinguishing characteristics of different hospice agencies. And agencies may provide individual aspects of care that go above and beyond what is required of them by law. For instance, some agencies have the ability to carve out insurance clauses for certain services whereby they broaden the scope of care that hospice is able to provide. Adjunctive services such as music therapy or massage may be provided by some hospice agencies as well.

Once the family has decided on the hospice benefit, the family signs consent for the patient. Of course, if a patient has the capacity to make his own decisions, he will sign his own consent, allowing for a nurse to come and evaluate the patient. In some cases, explanation of benefits may be done by the same nurse who will do the evaluation. The nurse will evaluate the patient's physical condition and prognosis based on a physical assessment of the patient, and a review of the patient's medical history and any medical records provided by previous medical providers. This is a standard process to determine whether or not the patient is eligible to receive the hospice benefit. If the patient is eligible to receive the hospice benefit and has signed consent, then the patient will be admitted as a patient of that hospice agency and services will begin immediately.

ADMISSION TO HOSPICE

Usually, at the time of admission, the nurse will provide the family with some type of "home chart", usually a binder or folder. This can be a way that the interdisciplinary team communicates with each other (though they will do this by phone and in person as well). It also serves as an informal record of medication administration, vital signs log, and a record of who visited a patient and when. You'll want to keep this chart available for the staff when they visit.

Hospices are able to provide a wide range of durable medical equipment such as a hospital bed, bedside commode, shower chair and oxygen equipment. These items are provided as needed and for the duration of services. The cost of equipment is usually covered by the hospice agency as part of the hospice benefit.

The nurse will order a standard set of medications called a "comfort kit". These are sometimes referred to as "e-kits".

The "e" stands for emergency. I'm not a fan of this term because in making the hospice decision, we have to develop a new paradigm. We are providing comfort care at the end of life. Hospice patients and families sometimes have urgent needs, but rarely have a true hospice-related emergency.

Usually, the comfort kit has a small quantity each of 5 or 6 different medications to help control some common symptoms at the end of life. These symptoms include nausea, constipation, pain, fever, anxiety, and agitation. Usually, these medications will come in a single container. Families are commonly instructed to "put this box in the refrigerator and forget about it" until they are instructed to use it by the hospice nurse. The hospice nurse should, however, go over the individual medications with you so that you have seen them at least once, and know basically how each medication works and when and how it should be used.

CERTIFICATION OF TERMINAL ILLNESS

In order for a patient to be admitted to hospice, it is required that two physicians certify the terminal illness, indicating a prognosis, or life expectancy of six months or less. This usually occurs when the patient's primary care provider or hospital physician writes the initial order for a hospice evaluation. Subsequently, the medical director for the hospice approves the clinical status of the patient. This happens by conference with the evaluating registered nurse and review of medical records. It is usually not necessary for the hospice medical director to visit the patient face to face upon the initial certification. It's important to note that there is no responsibility here for the patient or family other than providing clinicians with the patient's medical history when necessary. This section is included so that you can understand how hospice works and what might be happening behind the scenes.

90-DAY BENEFIT PERIODS

The first time a patient is admitted to hospice and certified to have a terminal illness they will receive a 90-day benefit period from Centers for Medicare and Medicaid Services. In the two weeks prior to the end of this 90 days, the registered nurse case manager will perform an assessment in order to certify that the patient continues to be eligible to receive the hospice benefit. This examination won't look any different than the nurse's routine weekly visit. Patients receiving hospice for the first time are generally eligible for two 90-day benefit periods.

60-DAY BENEFIT PERIODS

After the initial two 90-day benefit periods, the patient must be recertified by the registered nurse and a physician or nurse practitioner for a period of 60 days, by a face-to-face encounter. This process is repeated every 60 days with unlimited benefit periods possible, as long as the patient continues to decline thereby being considered eligible to continue to receive the hospice benefit.

Each time a patient is recertified, it means that the clinical team believes that the patient continues to have a life expectancy of 6 months or less, based on the normal progression of the disease.

DEATH

At the time of death, the hospice agency is notified by the family or caregivers. If the death occurs at a facility, the facility will notify the hospice. In the event the family is not present, the family may be notified by the facility or the hospice agency. Depending on the jurisdiction, a nurse will visit and make the official pronouncement of death. In some jurisdictions, or in specific, complex cases, it is necessary for the coroner or medical examiner to be notified. Also, the local public policy may require the sheriff's office or local police officers to attend the death as well. The hospice agency can also provide psychological and social support in the form of chaplains, social workers and music therapists for the benefit of the family and caregivers. After the nurse verifies the death, the hospice agency will report the death to the funeral home chosen by the family. The funeral home will then dispatch a car to pick up the body of the loved one.

The death of a hospice patient is not an emergency. Hospice agencies are respectful of various cultural beliefs and rituals at the time of death and immediately following. With this in mind, some facilities have specific policies and procedures surrounding the timely collection of a patient's remains. Furthermore, there may be local public policies guiding this procedure as well.

If you have specific cultural requirements with regard to preparation and collection of the remains of your loved one, you should communicate these needs early with your hospice team. This will help ensure a smooth and satisfactory process for everyone involved.

FAMILY BEREAVEMENT CARE

The psychological and social support team from the hospice agency will continue to be available to provide care and grief counseling and support to anyone whose life was touched by the deceased patient. Ask your agency for details about their bereavement program.

SECTION IV

THE HOSPICE TEAM

We're in This Together

Once a patient is admitted to the hospice agency, they will immediately be under the care of the interdisciplinary team including the Hospice Medical Director, Registered Nurse, Social Worker, Chaplain, Pharmacist and the Home Health Aide. Other services that are available may include Music Therapy, Massage Therapy, Dietitian, and Volunteers. This section deals with the professional functions of each member of the interdisciplinary team but let's be clear that the professionals partner with the family and friends as part of the care team in a supporting role. The hospice team directs and manages end-of-life care. They guide and teach and even provide direct care, but the responsibility for providing the majority of care lies with the family if the patient remains at home, or with the facility staff if the patient resides in a facility.

FAMILY AND FRIENDS

When I'm sick with a sore throat or the flu, I usually try to do my family a favor by staying in my room so that I don't expose them. But after a couple of days of isolation, I start to have very conscious thoughts of missing even the most casual interactions with my family. I crave having my wife sitting beside me and putting her hand on my shoulder. I actively miss hearing my kids laugh and tell me their stories, or showing me their latest project.

Sometimes after I've been sick and isolated, my emotional reservoir is drained, and it takes a concerted effort to refill it through reestablishing a connection with my family.

So many terminally ill patients are bedbound and confined to their homes or even sometimes a single room that they crave interaction and even a physical touch from someone they love.

On the other side of that coin is the family who is scared of what they don't know or understand about what is happening. They don't know what's okay to say or do. This trepidation and uncertainty sadly leads all too often to a paralysis and interactions are minimized or worse; abandoned altogether.

I admired a buddy of mine once. We had a mutual friend with ALS, also known as Lou Gehrig's disease, a terminal condition but one which is first utterly debilitating. In ALS there is a progressive death of the nerves that operate voluntary muscle. Our friend was confined to a wheelchair, totally dependent on her family for all of her basic needs. She wasn't able to talk or move at all. She did, however, retain enough movement in her right arm to operate the joystick of her motorized wheelchair.

As she rolled her wheelchair into church one week, she came to a bank of chairs with a full head of steam and made a hard right. I did a double take from down the aisle, seeing the potential catastrophe as she seemed on track to plow into a group of men standing in a circle talking. She weaved right again to thread the needle between the men and the front row of chairs. It all happened so fast. Then, sure enough, as she passed the group, my buddy yelled out in pain and recoiled. To everyone's horror, he was hopping up and down clutching his left foot. Our friend in the wheelchair, understanding what had happened stopped. She wasn't able to help, or even offer an apology. She just stopped as if to acknowledge her foul, when at the height of the intensity of the moment, while everyone was still processing what had happened, with perfect timing, my buddy stopped and smiled. He leaned down and with a pat on her shoulder said "I'm just kidding".

I'm not recommending that you mimic my buddy the next time you encounter a wheelchair. He had the right personality and the right relationship with our friend to execute a joke like this. But I tell the story because I was struck by his ease with her when so many people were reticent to interact with her at all. I was also struck by the expressions on her face. She seemed so appreciative that he just treated her like he would treat everyone else.

Sometimes the ability of your loved one to interact in ways that you are used to changes. But they are still the same person, and your history with them has not changed. The foundation of your relationship has not changed. Sometimes their ability to interact with you changes and can even cease altogether, but even so, their need for you to interact with them has not changed at all. This is true for those with memory loss, those who have become non-verbal, those who seem unconscious or are unresponsive, those who are in pain, those who are bed-bound, and those who are confined to a wheelchair.

It's okay to ask how someone is feeling and how things are going with their care. These topics don't need to be belabored, but they are not taboo either. You will not be 'reminding' them that they are sick.

It's also okay to talk about what's going on in your life. Talk about whatever you normally talk about. It doesn't need to be awkward or uncomfortable or unnatural. In fact, now more than ever, your loved one needs to have a very normal, familiar interaction with you. The same as you've always had.

It's okay, and even necessary to touch, talk and sing to your loved one—as long as whatever you're doing is consistent with the relationship you've always had.

Be you friend or family, you are a major component of the care team. Your involvement can have a profoundly positive impact on the end of life experience.

Meet The Professionals

PHYSICIAN

Hospices always have a medical director who is a licensed physician and may have associate physicians as well. The physician is the director of care and will be available to the hospice staff 24 hours per day. Hospice doctors work closely with the Registered Nurse Case Manager and the Interdisciplinary Team. They certify the hospice eligibility for each patient, and direct care by writing any necessary physician orders for medications and other parts of the plan of care.

REGISTERED NURSE

The RN is usually the case manager and acts as the Hub through which all other disciplines care for the patient. The nurse has direct lines of communication with the hospice medical director who is a physician, licensed to practice medicine and who may or may not hold hospice and palliative certification(s). Typically the nurse does not have to wait or go through a call center or answering service in order to communicate with the hospice physician which is a common practice in hospitals. This is important because hospice patients and their diseases have dynamic processes that require a close working relationship between the doctor and the nurse. The nurse also works closely with the social worker and is able to elicit their help when families need direction or aid with community resources such as placement in a facility, certain legal forms, government applications and even counseling when necessary.

SOCIAL WORKER

Often people are alarmed when they hear the term social worker because they associate it with something negative or with Child or Adult Protective Services when the state is intervening in someone's life, perhaps without invitation. But in hospice, the social worker is a valuable resource. They are required to have the highest level of training and licensure. They're capable of helping navigate through red tape such as might be found at The Veteran's Administration, Social Security, skilled nursing facilities, and contracts for respite care. They are also well qualified to counsel patients and their families regarding grief and loss and other psychosocial issues. Typically, the social worker will help guide a family in making final arrangements as well. It is true that all healthcare providers are required to report suspected abuse or neglect. But such a rare event should not be considered the social worker's normal function.

CHAPLAIN

Chaplains are also universally provided by hospice agencies and are available for psychosocial support and are well-versed and trained in counseling, specifically in the areas of grief and bereavement. While chaplains traditionally have personal religious views and preferences, they tend to practice in a non-denominational manner.

Sometimes, when asked about chaplain services, patients or families shrink. They assume that chaplains are only there to provide last rites. The truth is, chaplains are a big part of the overall support to you and your family that is offered by the hospice agency. They may also be able to help with community resources such as contacting a catholic priest to provide last rites, when necessary. Their services can be invaluable in grief counseling especially, for example, where difficult cases involving children are concerned. But you should know that just because the patient or family may not be religious, doesn't mean that the chaplain won't be of value. Chaplains are usually happy to provide non-religious support if that is warranted.

MUSIC THERAPIST

Some hospice agencies provide music therapy. You may hear them referred to as the "music lady" or the "guitar man". People commonly misunderstand them to be strictly for the patient's entertainment. The truth is that music therapists are bona fide therapists, board certified, and can be extremely therapeutic clinically and valuable in symptom control.

Music therapists work, in part, on what is known as the "Iso Principle" which is professional jargon meaning they can meet a patient where they are physiologically and use the power of music to manipulate physiological processes such as respiratory rate, anxiety and pain. They can be so effective that in some cases symptoms can be managed without medications. This is a good example of a non-pharmacological intervention mentioned earlier in this book.

HOME HEALTH AIDE

Home Health Aides are certified nursing assistants who work in a home care setting. Home Health Aides are not clinicians, but those who choose to work in hospice are often very experienced and have a great deal of knowledge and know-how. They are great resources both for providing bedside care and in teaching caregivers and families to care for bed bound patients. They can also teach techniques that are used in caring for patients who have lost mobility or who require feeding or other activities of daily living.

Sometimes caregivers are under the mistaken impression that home health aides will come and be with the patient around the clock. This is not accurate. Home Health Aides are given a specific plan of care by the registered nurse case manager. For instance, the care plan for a patient may include bathing the patient either in the shower or by bed bath. In the case of bed-bound patients, the care plan may include fingernail hygiene and trimming. It may also include linen changes or similar tasks. The Home Health Aide will be scheduled to do these tasks anywhere from 1 to 5 times per week. The aide will typically coordinate the time with the family or caregivers. When the Home Health Aide arrives at the bedside, they will go about completing the tasks on the care plan in an efficient manner, and when the tasks are complete, the aide will leave the home.

VOLUNTEERS

Volunteers are required by the Centers for Medicare and Medicaid Services to be provided by hospice agencies. Therefore, every hospice agency actively recruits volunteers for hospice patients.

Volunteers are generally utilized to provide companionship to a hospice patient. This can be extremely valuable where a patient's friends and/or family support system is limited either in size or capacity to provide emotional support to a patient. However, volunteers are not able to provide any type of hands-on care for patients such as bathing or changing diapers. Sometimes family members who need a break are tempted to utilize volunteers to sit with a patient while they run errands. While in some circumstances this might be permissible and may be arranged, it is not advisable because volunteers are not able to provide hands-on care. Hospice does provide respite care for caregivers who need a break. For more information on respite care see the chapter entitled Levels of Care in Section II.

It is worthwhile to remember that volunteers are giving of their own time and resources to serve the community. As such, they hold jobs and attend school, and have other responsibilities that may limit their availability.

SECTION V

WHAT DOES IT LOOK LIKE WHEN MY LOVED ONE IS DYING?

Decline

D ecline is a natural part of the end of life. It is something that is watched very closely by the hospice team. For ease of explanation, I have divided it into two categories: Acute decline, and chronic decline.

ACUTE DECLINE

Some disease processes by their nature have unpredictable and sometimes sudden outcomes. Unfortunately, the difficult truth is that it is possible for patients who have cardiovascular type diseases such as stroke or heart failure to be alert and oriented and interactive one moment, and gone the next. In cases where these or similar diseases are present, it is beneficial for patients to receive the hospice benefit earlier on in the process of decline. Being admitted to hospice earlier allows the clinical staff to obtain a baseline assessment of the patient which will allow for quicker response in the event of a more rapid decline. To put this in terms of a formula, earlier hospice facilitates a better patient-clinician relationship which equals better, faster care.

CHRONIC DECLINE

In other disease processes such as Alzheimer's Dementia, or Parkinson's Disease, patients tend to have a more predictable, slower decline. In these types of conditions, your hospice team can often give more specific guidance as to how a disease is progressing and what to expect next. It is beyond the scope of this book to give comprehensive disease-specific decline progressions.

Transition

Generally, after a disease has been identified as being in its final stage, there is an intermediate period between the general decline and the final phase of life when a patient is actively dying. This intermediate period is called Transition. Although it is important to remember that everyone is different and no two death experiences are alike, transition is usually marked with specific phenomena as described below, which signal the final decline and the "Transition to the Active Dying Phase". This is a phase rather than a specific period of time. Because people are all so different, this phase is different for everyone. It may only last a short time like a few days, or it may be prolonged for a period of weeks.

As we delve into the various signs that the end of life is near, it should be noted that most patients experience one or more of the following. There are also symptoms, not included in this list, like nausea, and constipation that are also common at the end of life. These symptoms are not included in this list because they are not necessarily caused by the dying process itself and should be assessed by your hospice team.

It should also be understood that it is important to look at trends. Be careful not to assume that because your loved one is nauseated, or takes an extra nap one time, that this means they are imminently dying. It could simply be that they ate something that didn't agree with them, or that they hadn't slept well the night before.

If you are caring for a hospice patient in any capacity, including just visiting intermittently, one of your primary responsibilities is to create and maintain a panic-free zone. Don't make a rash judgement based on one momentary observation.

WITHDRAWAL

When approaching the natural end of life, people tend to become less social. If they continue to have good cognitive function, they may become more introspective. They may become less interested in hobbies or television.

This natural, normal withdrawal can cause caregivers to react in various ways. Sometimes, without realizing the genesis of this withdrawal, caregivers believe that they can or should pull the patient out of it by forcing them to be in social situations.

On the other hand, though also rooted in failing to recognize the purpose of the withdrawal, some caregivers are more prone to allowing it to become personally offensive to them. It hurts their feelings because they feel as though they are being rejected or shunned by their loved one.

Either of these common reactions of caregivers may be disruptive to the patient's intellectual and emotional processing of their own mortality which is so valuable for a positive end of life experience.

INCREASED SLEEP

There is plenty of research, and much has been said about the brain's ability to continue to work on problems while the body sleeps. Even without research, society has long reflected this understanding in its colloquial speech. When facing tough decisions or circumstances, we say "Why don't you sleep on it?", or "Let me sleep on that and I'll get back to you".

Sleep is an important part of the dying process too. It may well contribute to the mental and emotional processing of the end of life and mortality.

No doubt, there is a physiological component as well. As organs and systems begin to function less efficiently and to slow down, sleep helps to conserve and manage energy and other physiological resources and processes.

Sleep is a comfortable state. Increasing sleep for someone who is at or nearing the end of life is normal and beneficial. Similarly to withdrawal, caregivers often try to intervene when they sense increasing sleep of their loved one. They may believe that the patient needs to get up and around in order to maintain their health. They may believe that the patient's health is declining because they are sleeping so much. This is incorrect, as the opposite is true at the natural end of life. Caregivers needn't worry about increasing sleep at the end of life and it is not necessary to intervene.

UNFINISHED BUSINESS

I once had a patient to whom I made weekly visits. Her daughter who was also elderly was her primary caregiver. This patient was totally bed-bound. Her limbs were contracted, meaning that they were fixed in a bent or flexed position. She ate a few bites of applesauce a couple of times a day. Her skin was pale and stretched thinly over her bones. The first time I saw her, she appeared to be close to death. I made my visit consistently week by week for months on end. At each visit, the patient's daughter would say "Well I can't believe she's still here. I don't know what she's waiting for". This went on week after week after week. At first blush, the daughter's comments seemed somewhat detached and out of place. But the fact was that she was simply exhausted from providing excellent, diligent and respectful care. The patient's grandson whom she had raised, had been incarcerated in a state prison. But his time had been served, and he was scheduled to be paroled. When he finally did get his release, he returned home to see his bed bound, now nonverbal grandmother lying quietly in a hospital bed in her room. Her daughter would tell me later that they had a very happy reunion in which she actually spoke a few words. She died the next day.

Despite being bed bound and nonverbal; totally immobile; my patient was somehow aware that her grandson would come home, and it seemed to me that she maintained the will to live in order to see that day. I've seen this unfinished business phenomenon over and over in my career.

This example of the will to live and unfinished business also is manifested in different ways. A chaplain once told me that a patient of hers confessed a crime he committed as a child--the nature of which she said she would "never communicate to another living soul". She continued to work with him and to help him understand spiritually that if he had repented of his sin that he indeed would be forgiven. It wasn't until he accepted that as fact that he was able to let go and he subsequently transitioned and died.

Still, others have no clear unfinished business and yet continue to hang on to life. It's common in these situations for families and caregivers to become exhausted in taking care of their loved one. Very often families will ask "Why are they still hanging on?" I usually answer with the statement that everyone is different and that personality often plays a role in a person's will to live. Then I might start to probe: "I don't know if he was a stubborn kind of person, but that often has an influence on how things progress..." Lots of times people will smile at a prompt like this, and you can see them begin to reminisce, and they often make a comment like, "Oh, Dad is stubborn alright. He always paddled his own canoe".

One last consideration is the notion that sometimes patients will hang on until they become confident that their survivors will be okay. There may be specific scenarios that they are worried about, or it may be more general. In any case it's often helpful, provided you can do so genuinely, to reassure your loved one that you are okay and that it's okay for them to go. This is called giving permission. Giving permission to a loved one to die is a fulfillment of the hospice philosophy. It can be both compassionate to the patient, and cathartic for the survivor.

Actively Dying

After transitioning, patients move into the Actively Dying phase. On average this lasts anywhere from one to seven days, with personality and other psychological or social issues being a factor. At the outside, I have seen this Actively Dying phase last up to 3 weeks. This chapter is designed to help you understand what to expect at the very end of life.

DECREASED ORAL INTAKE

At the end of life, it should be expected that the patient will have a decreased amount of oral intake both in the form of solid food and liquid. This may be associated with a decrease in appetite (the desire to eat and drink). In chronic conditions, this may be a trend over a long period of time with small incremental decreases in both appetite and intake. In the active dying phase, however, some patients may take in very small amounts of food, as in one or two small bites daily and minimal sips of fluid. But for the majority of patients actively dying, oral intake is reduced to zero. This is okay! And you should not feel like you are starving your loved one to death. For more on this, see the chapter entitled "Am I Starving My Loved One to Death?" on page 85.

DECREASED RESPONSIVENESS

At the end of life, patients often become less responsive. This is a general change in their consciousness. It may start with the patient sleeping more. This may simply mean longer nights at first, followed by taking more frequent naps during the day. These stages often occur slowly over all three phases of decline. Eventually, patients may sleep more than 22 hours per day. In the Actively Dying phase, it would not be uncommon for patients to sleep around the clock, except for being woken up for feeding or some similar activity of daily living. Sometimes patients will be able to be aroused, and while awake they are alert and oriented. Others do not respond to stimuli. This is not to say that they have no awareness of their surroundings, so it is important for loved ones to continue to be with them, talk to them, sing to them and touch them.

CHANGES IN BREATHING

Breathing patterns change at the end of life. In some disease processes such as Heart Failure or Chronic Obstructive Pulmonary

Disease, a patient's breathing pattern may already be abnormal. But in other disease processes, as life draws to a close, there can be significant changes in respiratory rate, depth and pattern or rhythm. Breathing may become rapid or slow, shallow or deep. This pattern can be very dynamic, changing from moment to moment. These changes can be somewhat disconcerting to caregivers and loved ones at the bedside. But these changes are a normal part of the dying process. Also at the end of life, the upper airway can become moist with secretions. This can cause the act of breathing to become quite noisy, making a gurgling sound. This sound is sometimes called the "death rattle". In spite of its ominous name, usually at this point the patient has become less responsive and has a decreased gag reflex, so the patient is comfortable. Nevertheless, this wetness can be treated with a medication that helps to dry out those secretions.

URINE CHANGES

As a patient approaches the end of life, their body systems begin to slow down, and there are often changes in urination. This usually means a decrease in urine output, meaning the patient is not urinating as frequently as they once were, or as might be considered normal. Also, urine usually changes color to become quite dark, even tea colored. That's because it is concentrated. With decreased fluid intake, patients become a little bit more dehydrated. This is combined with the fact that the kidneys, which make urine, begin to function less efficiently. This reduces the volume and frequency of urination. These are not problems for the patient who is actively dying. There is no discomfort associated with concentrated or decreased urine production at the very end of life.

SKIN CHANGES, MOTTLING

Changes also occur to the skin. This is because as life draws to an end, body systems are starting to change, to slow down, and to be less efficient. As a normal part of the dying process, circulation is no longer as efficient. This can cause the skin to take on a pale quality, and as mentioned in the section on urination, dehydration can change the appearance and texture of the skin so that it might appear to be a bit dry or waxy. The circulatory changes may result in a patient's extremities being cool to the touch. There can also be other color changes. If you have ever gotten out of a cold pool or lake, you might have noticed that there was a purple or blue marbling effect to your skin. This is caused by contraction or constriction of the blood vessels. During the dying process, the body naturally constricts the blood vessels in order to push blood to the body's core (the trunk, rather than the extremities), or vital organs which reside in the torso. This blue or purple marbling effect is called mottling. Mottling is a "sign" rather than a symptom. There's no discomfort to the patient.

As organs begin to slow down, the liver becomes less efficient. Subsequently, the body can take on a slightly yellow color known as jaundice. Jaundice also has no bearing on the comfort of a patient.

VITAL SIGNS CHANGES

Often during a process of decline families and caregivers become accustomed to taking blood pressure and temperature and other vital signs. Many times, this has been necessary in order to medicate a patient properly. In the stage of active dying, however, the body is working very hard to regulate all of the changes that are going on. For this reason, vital signs become less important because they give us less information. They become inadequate in helping us direct care.

Vital signs at the very end of life can be high one moment, and low the next. They can be at both ends of the spectrum from one moment to the next. So whereas at one time it made sense to monitor the vital signs or blood pressure, now that we know that the patient is actively dying, we understand that the blood pressure can be in the 160s one moment and in the nineties or even lower the next.

Sometimes caregivers become emotionally attached to procedural things like checking blood pressure or giving medications because it gives them the sense that they are 'doing something'. Fluctuating vital signs at the very end of life do not necessarily need to be treated medically, so it is important for families to be careful not to become obsessed with the numbers or the procedures. Rather, I instruct my patients' families to take a step back and look at their loved one's condition as a whole.

The primary question to ask yourself during this stage is "Do they look comfortable?" The patient's comfort becomes the preeminent concern at this stage of life because we understand that we cannot reverse the event of natural death. While the body's temperature may reach 100 or 101degrees, this is frequently momentary and does not indicate an infection. It simply may not need to be treated.

Very frequently the temperature will be high one moment and then back down to normal or even below normal a short time later. This is where I ask families to ask the question, "Are they comfortable?" If the patient's face is relaxed, not grimacing, and they're not sweating, then we assume that they're comfortable and no intervention is needed. On the other hand, if a patient has a furrowed brow, with a high temperature and is sweating, we can assume that temperature is high enough to cause the patient to be uncomfortable requiring an intervention such as giving a fever-reducing medicine or other non-pharmacological interventions.

The main idea is to start from the question of comfort and to not rely on diagnostic tools and numbers. You will be less stressed, and your loved one will be more comfortable.

VISIONS

Patients nearing the end of life often report having visions. In some cases, patients report seeing religious figures gesturing to come to them. In other cases, patients will talk to people who have already died. Still, more will talk to people from their past such as childhood friends. It's not uncommon for people to have conversations with somebody or call out names of people whom the family knows nothing about and often this can be traced back to childhood friends or other figures from a patient's youth.

RESTLESSNESS, ANXIETY AND AGITATION

Sometimes at this stage, there is anxiety or even agitation. These words can elicit a whole range of thoughts, but in the context of end-of-life, there are more specific definitions. I once asked a family caregiver over the phone if her Mom was agitated. She said "No, she's not agitated" and then went on to describe exactly what hospice clinicians would call agitation. I realized later that this particular patient had been an easily "agitated" person throughout her life. So when I asked if she was agitated, the caregiver pictured her short-tempered, irritated mother that she'd known from childhood, and said: "No, she's not agitated."

End-of-life anxiety and agitation can range from mild restlessness to trying to climb out of bed over the bedrails.

Mild restlessness might be as simple as a patient not being able to find a comfortable position, or constantly pulling or tugging at the bed sheets or their clothing. They may even try to take their clothes off.

Sometimes, patients will make repeated statements. "Let's go home…Let's go home…Let's go home". Other common statements are "Let's go", "Come on", and "Help me".

In more extreme cases, patients might cry out, scream or even become physically combative. It's important for caregivers to know that while not every patient will have these symptoms, when they do, it is normal and not personal. It's also important to know that the hospice team is adept at recognizing and treating these symptoms.

As a caregiver, you should remember that the environment can impact a patient's comfort and anxiety. Too many people in the room, bright lights, loud conversation, and televisions are a few sources of stimulation that may increase or exacerbate anxiety and agitation. On the other hand, dim light, soft talking, singing, or soft music may serve to reduce anxiety and agitation.

RALLY

This section should serve as both encouragement and a word of caution.

Patients at the end of life, and especially in the actively dying stage may have what's commonly called a rally. More crudely, but perhaps more accurately, it is sometimes called "the last hoorah". You may watch a loved one for days or weeks, become progressively more withdrawn from social situations, followed by increasing sleep and maybe even becoming completely unresponsive. It is not uncommon for a patient in this phase to wake up, have a lucid conversation with their surrounding loved ones, and even ask for something to eat. This type of rally is a clear one, but rallies take different forms. Often they are much more subtle, leaving even the professionals questioning whether the patient is truly having a rally. Sometimes it is after the fact when the realization is made that the patient appeared to have had a rally.

My word of caution stems from several sad and similar scenarios that I have witnessed at the bedside. Families which are not aware of, or prepared for the rally, have mistaken the apparent rebound for a miracle or an inexplicable reversal of the disease, only to be overwhelmingly disappointed when their loved one becomes unresponsive again and dies a short time later. Please be aware of this phenomenon and understand that it is momentary. I've seen these moments last anywhere from a few minutes to a few days or more.

I believe the rally is a great gift for many patients and families whereby the patient and their loved ones are able to say goodbye and to share a special moment of closure. It should be understood however, that this phenomenon is not guaranteed to happen, and does not happen for every patient. It is included here so that you might recognize it if you see it. Knowing what it is may help you make the most of it.

Am I Starving My Loved One to Death?

The short answer to the title question of this chapter is no. When a patient has a terminal disease, the end of life comes with a general decline. If you were to do sequential calorie counts, you would most likely see that a patient in the final stage of life decreases their oral intake in a stepwise fashion. This happens because the body is no longer using the nutrition that it's taking in. The body appears to be somewhat self-regulating in this regard. This decrease in oral intake will continue throughout the disease process for the most part until patients reach the very end of life, at which time they may not be eating or drinking at all. Because it is woven into our culture that we feed people when we're taking care of them, we tend to make a direct association between food and well-being. When a patient is at the end of life, we have to change our paradigm.

Patients at the end of life are not dying because you are not feeding them. Rather, they are not eating because they are dying. This is an important distinction for caregivers to understand. Caregivers are often overcome with guilt because they cannot get a patient to eat or drink. This is not the fault of the caregiver, and in fact is a normal part of the process of death and dying. The rule of thumb for caregivers who are not certain whether a patient is hungry or would like to eat is to offer food, but not to force it. If a patient declines food, the caregiver should assume that the patient does not need it, and will not metabolize or process the food if they do take it. Forcing a patient to eat, who does not have an appetite, and who may not use the nutrition that he takes in, can create other problems.

Force-feeding or even overly encouraging someone to eat can complicate the overall care of that patient and their well-being. For instance, if a patient is forced or overly encouraged to eat, but his digestive tract is slowing down, this can create new problems such as constipation or nausea and vomiting. If a patient is overly encouraged or forced to drink fluids that their body will not or cannot process thoroughly, other problems may arise such as swelling. This swelling, called edema, can also put additional pressure on the heart and lungs. It may even cause the lungs to accumulate fluid, making a patient short of breath, fatigued and generally uncomfortable. Actually, for a patient who is at the very end of life and has become totally immobile or perhaps unresponsive, some dehydration can actually be beneficial. Dehydration at this point causes the skin to be a little bit tougher, which may provide a small defense for things like bed sores.

SECTION VI

DIFFICULT DECISIONS

CPR and Hollywood

I'm going to be very straight with you about a very difficult topic. Hollywood has done a great disservice to our culture when it comes to the reality of Cardio-Pulmonary Resuscitation (CPR). Episode after episode of shows like Baywatch, popular cop shows, and movies have perpetuated a false notion of CPR.

The scenario goes like this: There is a natural disaster or some other tragic event that renders someone lifeless. In the case of Baywatch, it might be a drowning. The hero swoops in at just the right time and performs CPR for an intense and riveting minute or two, at the end of which, the victim rolls over, coughs, spits out some water and then wakes up. Over the next few seconds, the victim becomes alert again, hugs their loved ones, thanks the hero, and walks off into the sunset. This scenario is persistently portrayed by Hollywood, and it is a farce. This is not a normal outcome of CPR, and it is not an accurate portrayal of the realities of this extremely invasive, aggressive procedure. Make no mistake, CPR is an effective life-saving procedure. But it is only effective for the right candidate. In some cases, CPR is simply inappropriate.

In the text that follows I will try to help you understand the different scenarios in which CPR is appropriate and also the type of scenarios in which it is not. In explaining this to my patients, I often use this hypothetical example of an athletic man, healthy, in his forties, playing in the city softball league who takes a line drive to the chest interrupting the electrical circuitry of his heart and causing it to stop beating. The same could be applied to a healthy adult woman involved in a car accident; she stops breathing, and her heart stops beating. These patients are ideal candidates for aggressive resuscitation using airway support, artificial breathing, and chest compressions. You'll note that both these scenarios have in common that each individual has a healthy, vibrant life, possibly has children or young family at home and they have the potential to return to a normal life after this event. For these victims, CPR is totally appropriate and recommended.

But let's change gears and look at those patients who have been referred to hospice by their physicians after having been diagnosed with a terminal illness for which there are no more curative treatment options. These patients are at the natural end of life. Medical science has done all that it understands to do to intervene, and has determined that it can do no more. It's at this point that some families and caregivers are driven very strongly by their desire to hold on to the life of their loved one and therefore insist on doing "everything in their power."

But this is a short-sighted view often born of ignorance and a romanticized, Hollywood concept of CPR.

CPR is ugly. Let's look at the timeline of the process of CPR and the activation of the Emergency Medical Response System. It might go something like this. When a family member or caregiver notices that a patient has stopped breathing and no longer has a pulse, they call 911. When CPR is done accurately, the chest wall is compressed two inches deep which puts enormous stress on the body, usually breaking ribs.

When the ambulance arrives, EMS personnel will take over the CPR. They will begin intense compressions. They will insert a plastic tube into the patient's airway and begin artificial respiration. They will start an I.V. and begin administering fluids and medications. Elderly, frail patients often do not survive CPR. The Emergency Medical Services crew will transfer the patient from the home onto a stretcher or gurney and into the ambulance where CPR will continue. If possible, paramedics will initiate defibrillation (electric shock) in an attempt to restart the electrical activity of the heart. The patient will eventually be transferred to the emergency room where CPR will continue. The ER physician will continue to attempt resuscitation, both with electrical defibrillation and with chemical methods.

If the patient is stabilized, from the ER, they will be transferred to an intensive care unit on an artificial breathing machine called a ventilator. It is possible for a patient to recover from this event. But recovery is a long and difficult road even for the healthiest patients.

Now let's go back to our scenarios in the case of the softball player or the lady in the accident. They both have reasonable, though not guaranteed, chances of survival and returning to their normal lives. And even if the chances are low, considering the potential, activation of the EMS system is recommended and optimistic. Not so with one who is dying a natural death.

Now let's look at the patient who has been diagnosed with a terminal disease and has a six-month prognosis. Their bodies are already in a weak and fragile state, and we know they are at the natural end of life. This brings us to the question "What is the goal of care?" Let's go back to the ICU where our loved one lies with newly broken ribs from CPR, a terminal diagnosis for which there is no medical intervention available or for which the patient has already decided against treatment. And now, predictably based on their terminal diagnosis, they have not responded well to resuscitation and are dependent upon artificial ventilation. At this point, the family and caregiver have a new and challenging decision to make: "Do we remove our loved one from life support?"

There are questions that we can ask to help us determine whether or not we should perform the seemingly heroic measures of medical resuscitation. "What are our goals of care?" "What is our desired outcome?" "If it becomes possible to take my loved one home after CPR, what is their potential to recover?" "What is the potential of my loved one to return to a normal life?" "What will their quality of life be after CPR?"

It's usually necessary to change our paradigm after our loved one has been diagnosed with a terminal disease. It is no longer one of emergency management, but one of allowing natural death.

The scenarios above are intended to be overly general to illustrate the difference between a patient or victim who has the potential to return to a normal life or at least acceptable quality of life, and one for whom CPR borders on abuse.

Ultimately the decision to resuscitate or to attempt to resuscitate a patient or a victim lies with the patient or the patient's surrogates. These decisions are almost always complex with many variables. But the decisions need to be made by the family, and everyone involved who is reasonably deemed to have a say in the matter needs to understand and agree with the plan. As much as possible, these decisions should be made in advance.

I have worked with patients and families who just could not accept the notion of allowing natural death. They believed that they had a duty to do everything that was in their power to save the life of their loved one, even when it was known to be futile. Some people simply have that need, and I make no judgment on them. For some, this is the way that they cope with the loss of their loved one.

If after reading this chapter you still feel that activating the emergency medical system for your terminally ill loved one is the best course of action or a course of action that you must follow, I'd still like to make one recommendation. I recommend getting the do-not-resuscitate form signed anyway. Signing the form in the home setting is a multi-step process that requires signatures from both a third-party unrelated witness and a physician. This process takes some time. If the patient stops breathing and ceases to have a heartbeat you can always activate the emergency medical system. This is true even if you have a do-not-resuscitate order in place signed by the family, signed by a witness and signed by the physician. A caregiver or patient may always exercise their right to revoke the do-not-resuscitate order.

On the other hand, if a family or patient decides that they no longer wish to have heroic measures or to activate the emergency medical system or to transfer to a hospital, it is very difficult and maybe impossible to get a do-not-resuscitate order signed in the moment of an event.

I have seen cases where extended family members who happened to be visiting the patient when they died, panicked and called 911 despite the family's wishes. CPR was then initiated, and the hospital transfer occurred because there was no do-not-resuscitate order in place. This can be a traumatic and painful experience for the family and the patient.

I recommend you gather your family now, have this discussion, difficult though it may be, and come to a consensus. This can save you and your family and your loved one a great deal of emotional and even physical stress as your loved one's life draws to an end.

Clarifying Goals of Care

CARING FOR A TERMINALLY ILL LOVED ONE AT HOME

In the ideal situation, most family caregivers prefer to keep their loved one at home throughout the process of death and dying. This is not always possible, and later in this chapter, we will discuss several options when home care is not possible and reasons why it may not be.

When you are determining to care for a loved one who is entering the final stages of life, you will inevitably face various challenges. If you are alone, what will you do when you have to go to the grocery store, or the bank, or run other types of errands? What if you become exhausted? Do you have someone that can stay with your loved one while you are getting some rest? There are unique safety concerns with seriously ill people living at home. These may be related to immobility or poor judgment as in the case of dementia.

When a patient becomes bed-bound and incontinent, this represents challenges. If you're not accustomed to caring for a bed bound patient your hospice nurse and home health aide can guide you and instruct you in techniques for turning a patient, bathing, changing diapers, and even changing linens while the patient is still in bed. While many of these tasks may sound daunting now, rest assured the hospice team is there to support you. Much of the work, such as bathing, can be done on a scheduled basis anywhere from 1 to 5 times a week by the home health aide, but you as the caregiver would still be responsible for taking care of the patient when the hospice aide is not there.

This is difficult work, and it can be emotionally and physically exhausting. At the same time, this is noble and rewarding work that enhances the relationship between you and your loved one. In my experience, families who care for their loved ones at home ultimately tend to cope better with their loss. This in part, is because they see up close and personally the changes in the condition of their loved one through the dying process and in turn, they gain a heightened awareness that the end of life is approaching which in many cases means an end to suffering.

There should be no shame felt in the relief that naturally comes with the death of a loved one after the family or caregiver has engaged in such meaningful care. Personally, I believe this relief is a gift from God and a natural reward for a job well done. There should also be no shame when circumstances dictate that a patient is placed in an assisted living or long-term care facility. Among the reasons that this may need to take place might be debility of the caregiver such as might be in the case of an elderly spouse. There may be emotional situations or family dynamics or aggregate living situations, or myriad other scenarios which simply prohibit at-home care.

In cases such as these, families have several options. I strongly recommend that you utilize the interdisciplinary team, namely the social worker and the nurse case manager in steering you toward the most appropriate option. Options include skilled nursing facilities which operate similarly to hospitals with nurses assigned to patients around the clock, and with attending physicians available by phone. Skilled nursing facilities are good options when skilled care is required. Your hospice team can help you determine such reasons.

Assisted living facilities are another option. Usually, though, this option requires that a patient posesses some level of independence. Assisted living facilities are not set up to provide any type of clinically skilled care. Caregivers at these facilities may provide wellness checks, meaning that they will peek into the patient's private apartment to see if they're ok. They might provide some level of incontinence care and hygiene. They provide room & board. They will, however, maintain a relationship with the hospice agency and will communicate when the patient or resident is in need.

A better and probably more appropriate option for hospice patients is a Board and Care Facility sometimes called a personal care home. These are small residential facilities that are usually discreet single-family dwelling style homes with a special license to care for a small number of residents. I like Personal Care Homes because the staff is usually adequate to care for the, on average, three to six residents that are living in the home. In these facilities, caregivers tend to have a closer relationship and bond with the residents. This means that they know the idiosyncrasies, habits, and needs of each individual resident.

Because of the nature of these facilities and their size, caregivers are much more in tune with the happenings of the residents. For instance, if a patient who is at high risk for falling tries to get off of the couch, usually there's a caregiver very close by that notices the impending accident and is able to intervene much more quickly than say in a skilled nursing facility or assisted living facility where patients are in a room with the door shut, out of sight.

The availability of these options must be assessed based on the patient's or family's financial resources and needs. Usually, the best person for this type of analysis in the interdisciplinary team is the social worker.

EXPECTATIONS

If you are faced with the hospice decision, one of the most important things for you to do is to clarify your own expectations. Have you done the internal work of processing this diagnosis and prognosis? If you don't believe the prognosis, and therefore don't believe that the end of life is near, then the benefit of hospice care will be significantly diminished. I believe that one of the biggest benefits of hospice care is the teaching and education that patients and families receive from the hospice team. If either the patient or the family is not accepting of the patient's diagnosis or prognosis, they will not be in a suitable frame of mind to receive the education and coaching that makes hospice helpful.

One of the primary goals of this book is to help you mentally and emotionally process your thoughts and feelings regarding the end of life and mortality in general. Given a long enough life, we will all have to process mortality at some point. The mistake most of us make is that we wait until we are facing a crisis before we give it the requisite thought.

In every aspect of life, we know, and may even preach to others, that planning ahead is wise and perhaps even our best insurance against failure. And yet, it would seem, that when it comes to processing mortality, we are all procrastinators.

I believe that those who engage in the difficult emotional work of mentally processing their own mortality and the mortality of their loved ones, early in adult life, and before facing a crisis, will be more capable of setting realistic expectations.

Before setting expectations for the hospice team and those around you, first determine what you are expecting from yourself and from this experience.

In addition to asking the big existential questions like Jim did in Two Journeys, ask yourself the more practical questions specific to the end of life. I recommend starting with a blank journal and writing in stream of consciousness. Writing your unfiltered thoughts can be cathartic, but it also helps solidify what you really think and feel. It helps you separate itinerant thoughts from actual feelings and beliefs. Don't use a keyboard for this. Write your thoughts out longhand. Don't edit while you write. You can analyze your thoughts later. Use these prompts and create your own:

What is my (or my loved one's) illness, or combination of illnesses?

What have the doctors said we should expect in the course of this illness?

Will this illness ultimately result in death? Why?

Is there anything medically that can be done to cure or reverse the disease?

Can life be prolonged? Would prolonging life increase the quality of life? Would prolonging life increase the value of life?

Would allowing natural death be appropriate and compassionate?

What do we need in the way of help?

Do I have the strength to care for my loved one at home, or should we consider placement in a facility? Now? In the future?

Should we sign an Allow-Natural-Death or Do-Not-Resuscitate order?

How will I handle the death experience?

Have we made funeral plans?

How do our cultural and religious beliefs apply to the end of life?

WHAT SHOULD I EXPECT FROM MY HOME HEALTH AIDE?

As mentioned in the section on the interdisciplinary team, the hospice aide will help the patient with activities of daily living which is primarily a function of hygiene such as bathing, oral care, and incontinence care. The home health aide will have a specific plan of care initiated by the registered nurse case manager, and the aide is not permitted to deviate from this plan of care. For this reason, it is recommended that the plan of care be developed with the patient and or family involvement. Once the home health aide has completed the day's plan of care, they will leave to move on to their next patient and should not be expected to provide care around the clock or even longer than is required to fulfill the plan of care. The home health aide will visit anywhere from 1 to 5 times per week depending on the needs of the patient. The frequency will be determined by the case manager and will be part of the plan of care. Changes to the frequency will require an official change to the care plan.

WHAT DOES THE SOCIAL WORKER DO?

Contrary to common public perception, the social worker is not there to interfere or take control of a family's or patient's affairs. Social Workers are valuable resources to the hospice community and can help in many ways from identifying resources to the family to grief or other types of counseling. The Social Worker will generally make an initial assessment of a patient's or family's needs within the first 5 business days of admission to hospice. From that point it will be determined what is needed by the patient or family and whether visits will be made only as needed or perhaps on a loose schedule, something like 1 to 3 times per month.

WHAT SHOULD I EXPECT FROM THE CHAPLAIN?

Chaplains in hospice have specific training in bereavement and grief counseling. They can help you process your thoughts and feelings with regard to the decline of your loved one. While chaplains are generally religious and most likely have a specific religion, they are fully capable of dealing with people in a non-denominational way. They are also able to help in other ways that might be religion or denomination specific. They tend to be willing to talk and counsel in spiritual, religious ways but also in broader more general ways as desired by the family. The chaplain will make an initial assessment after a patient is admitted to hospice and then will determine a visit frequency based on the needs of the patient or family. This can range anywhere from 1 to 4 times per month and can always be adjusted based on need.

WHAT SHOULD I EXPECT FROM THE VOLUNTEER SERVICES?

Volunteers provide companionship for patients. This can take the form of anything from just sitting quietly at the bedside, to talking and reminiscing, to playing games, singing songs or reading to the patient. Some hospices offer volunteers who provide pet therapy which has well-documented benefits, but the details of which are beyond the scope of this book. While it is required by the Centers for Medicare and Medicaid Services that hospice agencies provide volunteers, by definition the service of a volunteer is dependent upon that volunteer's availability. For this reason, volunteer schedules may be sporadic. It bears being mindful that volunteers are giving freely of their own time and resources to serve the hospice population. As far as I'm concerned, the world could use more people like them.

WHAT IS MY NURSE DOING AND THINKING ABOUT?

The registered nurse case manager is primarily concerned with the comfort of the patient and managing symptoms that impede comfort or quality of life. But the nurse is also concerned with the quality of life and the well-being of the family and caregivers, not only because the caregiver has a significant impact on the comfort of the patient, but also because supporting the family is part of the role of the hospice agency. As the case manager, the nurse is responsible for assessing the needs of patients and families that can be met by the other interdisciplinary team members and is also responsible for coordinating the care among the team, such as the Chaplain, Social Worker, Music Therapist, Home Health Aide, Volunteers, Dietitian, Physician, and Pharmacist. The nurse will be assessing for these needs, but don't be afraid to speak up if you feel you need one of the other services.

Also of note, is the fact that Registered Nurses are clinicians. As such, a lot of the work that they do has to do with the analysis of data. It may seem to laymen that the nurse is not 'doing' much when they make their visits. That's because a lot of the work they do happens in their brain. If a patient is progressing comfortably, there may not be a need for the nurse to do anything. But be sure, the nurse is doing more than you are able to observe. They are collecting data. They are analyzing any changes from what is considered to be the patient's normal condition, called the baseline. This is important so that they can recognize changes from the baseline which may require a change to the plan of care.

Nurses are also educators, and a big part of their job is to teach you what to expect of the disease process and how to care for your loved one. So don't be bashful about asking questions.

WILL I SEE A PHYSICIAN?

Hospices always have a Medical Director and sometimes associate Physicians, and Nurse Practitioners. The Centers for Medicare and Medicaid Services requires a provider face-to-face visit to certify the terminal illness prior to every 60-day benefit period. Some hospices are set up to have these Team Physicians or Medical Directors or Nurse Practitioners make symptom visits as needed.

But for the most part, your Nurse Case Manager is the Physician's eyes and ears. They are able to assess and report back to the Physician and collaborate with the Physician when symptoms need to be managed, but most experienced Registered Nurse Hospice Case Managers are able to manage most symptoms with the standing orders that are provided by the hospice Medical Director.

To simplify this, if a patient dies within the first 6 months of hospice care and has normal or average symptoms throughout their decline, they may not see a physician or provider other than the Registered Nurse. Conversely, if a patient is still receiving hospice care after the initial six-month benefit period, they must see a physician or nurse practitioner to certify that the patient continues to meet criteria to receive the hospice benefit. If you are interviewing hospices, ask the representative if the agency has physicians available to perform symptom visits if necessary.

Closing Thoughts

I've left a lot on the table. I'll take this line to reiterate that this book is not intended to be a substitute for the clinicians involved in your case. There is much left to be taught to you by your doctor and hospice team. If this book has fulfilled its intent, it has served merely to help you forge your perspective and to get you off on the right foot.

If a hospice diagnosis is new to you or someone you love, I strongly suggest that you find a way, if possible, to get out into a natural environment. Sit on a log in the woods or find a quiet place by a babbling brook. Nature is the best environment for gaining perspective. It's important to unplug and take time away from our technological devices. We live in a world so loud with noise from not only technology but from the frenetic nature of our lives, that we don't realize how conditioned to it we have become. We also don't realize the impediment that the busyness of our lives causes to our ability to process our thoughts. Too often we allow our technology to do our thinking for us.

It wasn't long ago that nearly all people lived some degree of agrarian life. They gathered eggs, slaughtered sheep and hunted to provide for their families. They sowed seed, and they grew crops. They cultivated baby plants into mature ones. They harvested. All of this served to provide a perspective of life and death. It was a constant reinforcement of the cycle of life.

I remember preparing for the funeral of a friend's baby who died at only three days old. I spent that morning in my garden. I can't quote science as to why this is so effective, but I felt renewed by the quiet, immovable forces of nature. I personally believe this is built in by the Creator of the universe. Tending my young lettuce plants that day, I had clarity; peace. The cycle of life was reinforced. My stress was dulled, my spirit was humbled. I had not been immunized from the full range of emotions that came with that event, but I was much more prepared to process my emotions with perspective.

Unplug. Schedule a time to shun the bustle of daily life for a while. Find a quiet spot in nature and dig deep. Wrestle with the ultimate questions of life. Ask "What is the purpose of life?" Think about life and death. Think about your life and memories. Ask "What is really important in life?" Spend some time thinking about mortality in general. Whose life have you celebrated? What made them worth celebrating? Think of the youngest person you know. Then think of the oldest person you know. Is length of life really paramount? Or is the quality of life and relationships more important? Are CPR, ER visits, ICU stays, tubes and wires and ventilators really the most appropriate courses of treatment?

These questions are difficult and direct. But they will help you to process your thoughts and to find perspective. This is hard work emotionally and spiritually, but it is necessary work that can pay large dividends in peace of mind.

If you decide to utilize hospice, take the time to interview hospice agencies. Choose an agency that is solely dedicated to the hospice/palliative care discipline, or at least one with a dedicated hospice division. Choose an agency with people and personalities with whom you click. Ask the doctor or hospital for recommendations.

When you have done the hard work of finding perspective and have peace with this diagnosis and prognosis, hospice can be extremely helpful in facilitating a warm and dignified end of life experience for all involved.

You can also take comfort in the knowledge that once this work of finding perspective has been done, daily life doesn't have to be all existential all the time. In fact, it shouldn't be. In Two Journeys, Jim spent a lot of time in the cleft of that tree planning his end of life work which was all about contributing to the lives of those he would leave behind. There was no magic in his plan; nothing spectacular. He planned things that for him were very much in the moment, but things which would provide lasting memories and feelings for his loved ones. He planned to take the grandkids fishing. He planned to embark on a quest with his wife to bake the perfect peach cobbler.

Jim's plan was elegant. The mental exercise of reviewing and affirming what he valued most had provided him with the existential perspective he needed to create the plan. But executing his work was both painless and enriching. These activities weren't heavy or existential at all. They were not threatening, or intimidating. They were easy. Easy and effective. He did normal things with those he loved, and in those acts, he was able to fully embrace the moments they shared. This is how you live your fullest life.

Now take a big, deep cleansing breath and relax. You're ready. You can move forward with confidence that you can play the role of either guest or host and have a rich and meaningful end of life experience.

MAKING THE HOSPICE DECISION

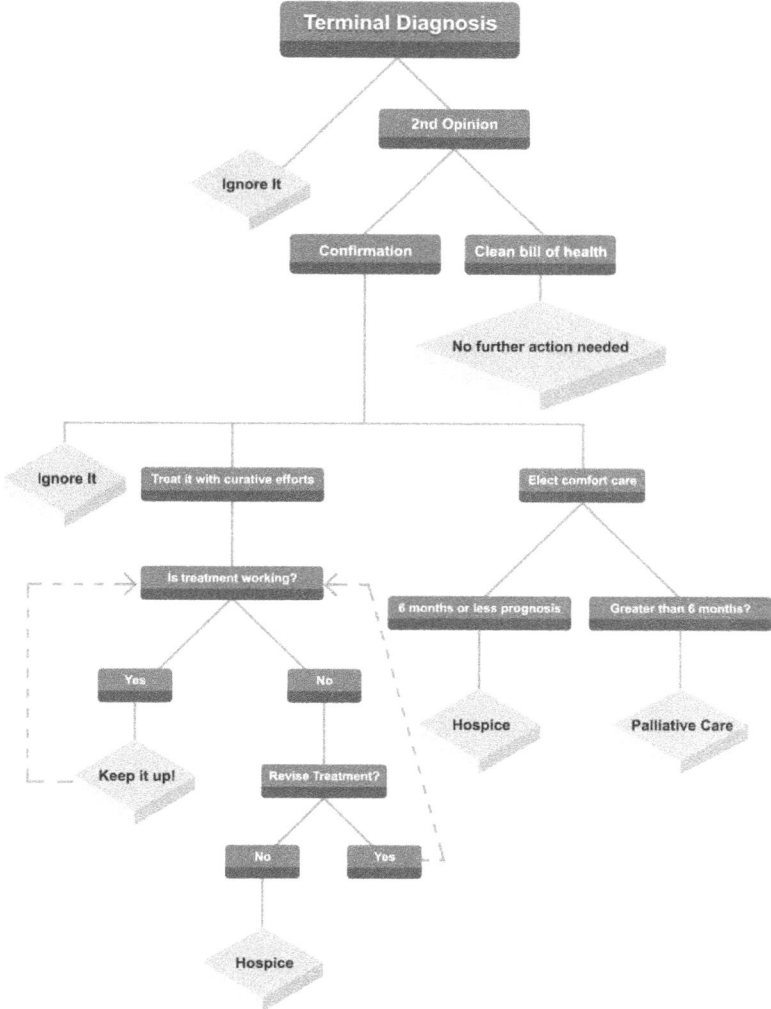

Figure 1

HospitiumUSA.org
RandalSalyer.com

Also available from Randal Salyer
and HospitiuM Books:

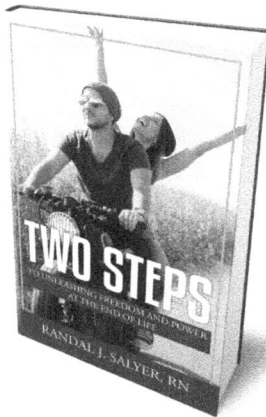

And Coming Soon:
Your Fullest Life
(a workbook)